Huh?

or

Hearing Utterances & Humor

or

Clarifying Hearing Loss & Hearing Aids: A Consumer's Guide

or

A Hearing Doctor Talks Shop

By Tonya L. LaLonde, Au.D.

Doctor of Audiology, Speaker

2009

email: tonyalalonde@gmail.com

Table of Contents

Why on earth I wrote this

Hello. I would like first to tell you who I am and why I wrote this book. I would like to, but I won't... just kidding. My name has been Tonya LaLonde for the last year, because that is how long I have been married to Steve, and I have been Mommy to Zachary (the most wonderful little boy ever) for the last five and a half of those and Kathleen (the most wonderful little girl ever) for the last nine months. Before that, it was Tonya Batterson, a little girl from a farm town in the Southwest corner of Michigan. I have been a Doctor of Audiology ("What?" is the traditional running joke that is no longer funny, by the way) for the past 9 years. My Bachelors of Science degree in Biomedicine was from Western Michigan University (go Broncos!), my Masters of Science degree in Audiology was from Bloomsburg University of Pennsylvania (bless their hearts), and my Doctor of Audiology degree is from the Arizona School of Health Sciences. I must tell you that my doctorate is a professional doctorate, which is different than medical school training to be a physician. I have worked with many, many wonderful patients (and some real stinkers) over the years in my own private Audiology clinic in Lakeland, Florida and several other places before that (PA, South FL, & CA) and since (Central Florida).

This book was written with every intention of helping my patients, potential patients, other people's patients, and especially you to understand everything you need to know about hearing loss, understanding loss, and hearing aids. This is important information because hearing problems are very prevalent in our society, and everyone is touched by it in some way- a relative, a coworker, a client, a peer, or (don't pass out now) maybe even you!

Now for my disclaimer... this is not a technical book, and I will be quoting as few people as possible on purpose. I am giving you information from my extensive experience, observations, and knowledge of this topic. I think of this book as a conversation, the way I would speak to you in my office, and the way I would want it presented to me.

One more thing... for those who do have a hearing loss, I would like to share with you that hearing loss is **not**- I repeat is most definitely **not**- age-specific. I have fit babies with hearing aids and people over 100. There is no reason to be ashamed of a hearing loss- it is common and imposes itself on everyone equally. It does not mean that you did something wrong (most of the time) or that you are in any way unintelligent (or more intelligent, for that matter). What you should be ashamed of is not doing something about it if you are able to. The hearing aids do not make you conspicuous. Asking "Huh?" most definitely does. You should be proud of yourself for acting positively for your overall health and happiness by obtaining help for your hearing loss. Well, I am a Mommy **and** a Doctor of Audiology... what do you expect?

Well, I hope you have clarity, entertainment, and understanding upon reading this little book. If you have further questions, feel free to contact me via email at tonyalalonde@gmail.com. There are certainly many other sources of information if you are more technologically minded and many other websites (disclaimer- do not believe everything you read on the web, as it is often unchecked and unreliable information) and books (see previous disclaimer) and Audiologists out there if you would like more information. My purpose, again, is not to be all-inclusive but to teach the basics that I know in a readable way. Enjoy!!

And remember one very important truth... before you insult another person, be sure that you first walk a mile in their shoes. That way, when you insult them, you'll be a mile away, and you'll have their shoes! ☺

Chapter 1
To Hear or Not To Hear

So there was a man who was convinced beyond all doubt that his wife had a hearing loss that she would not own up to. He was finally going to prove it and tell the doctor when they went to their annual check up the next day. So, as his wife is cooking dinner, he calls out in his normal voice from the next room, "Honey, what are we having today?" She doesn't respond. So, he gets a little closer and asks again. Four times he asked, each time getting closer. The fifth time he asked right behind her. Infuriated, she peels around on her heels and screams, "For the fifth time chicken!!" A common phenomenon? I think not. That is the reason these words are before you now. There is more to life than miscommunication and frustration. Time to dig in and live...

Absolutely, beyond a doubt, the most important fact I can convey to you about your hearing is that hearing and understanding are two **very** different things. The most common type of hearing loss does not affect the hearing but the understanding of speech. Hence, the most common complaint I hear in my practice is that, "I can hear fine but can't understand", or an alternate version of the same thing, "Everyone mumbles... if they would just speak clearly like you do I wouldn't have any problem at all." Yep. Every single day I hear one of those versions of the same thing or something very close to one of those versions.

I see you nodding and smiling, and I think I heard a few chuckles, because you know I'm right. Either you or someone you know has said the same thing at least once.

[Of course, all bets are off with children, because their most common complaint is not being able to hear (often accompanied by an earache, which should be checked out by an Audiologist or Physician as soon as possible).]

Why are hearing and understanding different? The biggest reason has to do with low frequency/pitch versus high frequency/pitch auditory information/sounds. You see, most of the vowel sounds ("a", "o", "u", etc.) and nasal sounds (like "m", "n", "l", etc.) of speech exist in the low pitches. Most of the discriminatory consonant sounds of speech (like "s", "t", "f", "th", "z", "h", etc.) exist in the high pitches.

What does that matter? Well, let me tell ya... if your hearing loss is primarily in the high pitches, but the low pitch hearing is okay, you will be able to hear those lower pitch speech sounds fine but **not** be able to hear the clarifying high pitch speech sounds well or at all. Thus, everyone would sound as though they are mumbling. And, of course, if someone is not ready to admit that they have a hearing loss, they will complain that people are, in fact, mumbling and that is the problem. "Kids these days don't know how to pronunciate... it's shameful," is what I'm likely to hear, or the related, "I can hear some voices fine, if they speak clearly, but not others," or even worse, "It's my wife's fault... she keeps talking to me as she walks away and no one would be able to hear her." While all that may be true some of the time, it most definitely not true all the time.

At this point, let me mention what a powerful force denial is. For those of you under the power of this disabling beast, please allow me to express from my heart sincerely that it takes a very strong person to admit that there might be something wrong with them... even something as simple as admitting a hearing loss. It's hard to deny a green nose, would be silly to try to deny a green nose, because it's obvious to everyone and you can look in the mirror and be reminded that you indeed have a green nose. A hearing loss and denial mechanisms are much more evasive, and often invisible, so it may be obvious to everyone else, but if the person themselves can't see it, it doesn't exist.

Again, let me point out that having a hearing loss does not mean that you are old... I diagnosed a 6-year-old today in my office. This little guy without even batting an eye said, "Okay," with a smile and thought it was pretty cool to wear hearing aids and was excited about picking out his favorite color (red). Having a hearing loss means **only** that you have a hearing loss. If you couldn't see so well anymore, you would have a vision loss and would wear glasses to fix it. If you are dehydrated, you have a water loss and you drink water to fix it. Don't over think it. Choose not to bring your own preconceptions or baggage into the mix. Leave it at the door. You have enough stress in your life. The aids these days are not your grandfather's aids. If you come to that realization, I applaud you for your intelligence and praise you for becoming proactive in your life and doing something rewarding for yourself and your loved ones!!!!

Now, for those of you with a loved one with who is in denial... until he (male pronoun for ease of writing only- don't take offense, men) decides to admit a hearing loss exists and until he is ready to be proactive in the treatment of that loss, there is absolutely nothing you can do to get him to do it. "You cannot push a rope," as my dad used to say. You can drag a horse to water, kicking and screaming with whips and threats and insinuations, but you certainly cannot make him drink. You can tease him, exclude him, manipulate him, and threaten to turn him into glue, you can even take away his social privileges, but if that stubborn horse still doesn't want to drink, he's not going to do it.

So if you are in that category, the only thing you can do to retain your sanity is admit that your loved one is as stubborn as a horse and has a hearing loss. In that light, there are compensations you can make yourself to make your life better. **Remember that the only person on the planet you can change is yourself**.

So, to keep your sanity, do **not** under **any** circumstances, try to speak to your loved one from another room. They can **not** understand you that way, so you will either become frustrated and want to throw something at him or be forced into the terrible position of having to repeat yourself, repeat yourself, sel**f, self, with an "f"!!!**

A second thing you can do is to always look at him to talk to him- don't have your back turned. This is not only so you can constantly be blowing kisses to him (tee hee), but also so he can read your lips. The closer you are to someone, the louder they hear you, but also the better they can watch your lip movements. I'll talk more about that in a minute.

Another thing you can do to alleviate your stress, is to turn off or pause the TV, radio, ipod, MP3 player, video game, computer volume, etc. or mute it **before** trying to carry on a meaningful conversation with him. This concept may also dictate to you that you go out to eat at quieter restaurants or go to quieter parties rather than loud restaurants or loud parties. Why does noise/music make things worse? Well, I'm glad you asked!

First, and most importantly, the nature of noise is that centered in the low and/or mid-frequencies/pitches. Why is that important? Well, the most common hearing losses affect the high frequencies more than the low frequencies, at least initially. Therefore, the low frequency noises around us drown out what we're good at (are heard well because of good or okay hearing in the low frequencies) and make you rely more heavily on the higher frequencies, which are not being heard properly anymore. So, you hear the noise but not the distinctions of speech, making it futile to try to communicate in noise without a lot of repetitions, lip reading, or other annoyances. Also, noises in restaurants and malls, etc. come in pretty loudly, and if he is used to hearing this quieter, the sound is overwhelming and bombarding, so a huge distraction. It would be like trying to have a casual conversation over coffee in your living room with a full grown elephant right in front of you... a little distraction, to say the least.

Speaking of lip reading for a moment now... I have a story to tell you. I had a lady patient- sweet little 93-year-old lady- come into my office about three years ago. I asked her, "What brings you into my office this fine day?" She looked at me quizzically and replied with the classic, "What was that?" So, understanding instantly what brought her into my office, with my infinite wisdom and education, I spoke louder in a lower pitch and repeated my question, "What brings you in today?" She gave me the sweetest smile and leaned over to pat my hand. Then she started fumbling through her purse and told me, "Wait a second, honey. Let me get my glasses on so I can hear you." And, like magic, once she put her eye aids on, her hearing did become significantly better!!! So, what does this tell us? I asked her, "How long have you been reading people's lips?" (In essence, I was asking when she first noticed she had a hearing loss.) She replied with a sweet laugh, "Oh, heavens, I don't know how to do that. It would be great if I could." It was all I could do not to laugh, because the dear sweet lady was already doing it better than anyone with formal training.

Our brains were created in such an intricate way that we are equipped to compensate somewhat for a hearing loss by automatically maximizing on our other senses and using visual cues (body language and lip movements) to get more information for interpretation. We are very social beings and this is one way we help keep ourselves in the conversation- the embodiment of socialization and thus humanity.

That little tangent was a nice segues into step three to make your life better. This is the toughest one, especially for really good helpers of their loved ones and those engaging in long-term helping habits. I warn you, this is hard. In all your love and understanding, knowing that you want to be helpful and show your loved one love and understanding, I implore and challenge you to stop enabling them.

Denial is a very secure island that someone has to choose to live on. Your stubborn loved one in denial is being assisted in his persistent denial by you. No doubt your intentions are commendable. But remember, all you can change is you. Generally, stubborn people- by that I mean those choosing to live on the island of denial- won't seek help if it's convenient for them not to. If **you** are their hearing aid, why do they need a device to do the same thing? Many people wait to come in until their loved ones are about to kill them if they have to repeat **one more word**!!! Think about it? Your helpfulness is keeping them content and informed, as you relay whatever is necessary to them. If, as an experiment, you were to decide just for 2 weeks, not to be their ears for them, what would happen?

Maybe, just maybe, you understand, they would be uncomfortable enough with missing out on life that they would be inspired to act on their behalf and attain the help they need. Disclaimer: tensions will be high on their part and frustration will be easily come by, but tensions on your part will be relieved as you will be doing the hearing for only one (you). Now, I know what some of you gentle folk are thinking... but I have to help my loved one. I am suggesting to you the possibility that you will be helping them more by showing some tough love than any other "help" you can give them. That is just food for thought... chew on it for a little while and see what tasty morsels can be digested, especially with the chocolate of less stress in your own life and the idea of less stress in theirs also once they come to grips with this.

No, if your loved one has decided to venture from the safe and secure island of denial, YEAH!!!!! And if you are that loved one who made the giant choice, GOOD FOR YOU!!! We have only now to talk about that hearing loss and what to do about it. Your hardest work is done! However, if that choice is not made yet, please rest assured that there is hope yet. Sometimes, having the right information helps, and the remainder of the book has it.

Chapter 2
That annoying ringing sound

Tinnitus is the little bugger. You can call it "tin-it-us" or "tin-I-tus"- from what I have read, for the most part, it makes absolutely no difference. A few would have it that if you use the latter, it is more indicative of being related to an infection. Regardless, this sound can take the form of a "ringing" or "crickets" or "high pitched sound" or "roaring" or "static" or "wind noise" or "thumping", etc. It can sound as if it's coming from the head or the environment or one ear or both, etc. It can come and go, change pitch, change volume, and most of the time be worse in quiet or at night. It is annoying in differing degrees to different people. It can start for no reason or as a result of a medical problem or medication or car accident or hearing loss or noise exposure, etc.

People often seek help for tinnitus from their doctor, thinking instantly that they have a brain tumor and are about to die. (Why is it our thoughts jump to that so eagerly anyway? What's that about?) Irregardless, the doctors, once they run a gamut of tests, will attempt to determine any medical cause for it. For instance, a "thumping" sound that keeps time with your heartbeat, even if it comes and goes, is often closely related to a blood pressure issue because the jugular vein runs very closely under the middle ear cavity. If, however, no medical cause can be pinpointed, often the patient will be told to get used to it and there's no treatment (which is false, by the way).

If there is no medical problem, the tinnitus may be due to noise exposure and/or hearing loss. In these cases, a hearing aid will help reduce or eliminate the perception of tinnitus by bringing in sounds to help mask it about 60% of the time. In 20% more of the cases, it will at least lessen it to the point of being okay with it. In the other 20% of the time, the patient does have to learn strategies to lessen it. There is help for these people through the American Tinnitus Association (a very good organization) and affiliated Audiologists who perform Tinnitus Retraining Therapy. I won't get into all that and how it works... it is discussed nicely in the American Tinnitus Association website, and you can contact them for more information.

If the tinnitus is not hearing loss related (or at least not yet, usually), one thing that helps get to sleep at night or relax is to have a noise maker on a peaceful sound (like the rain or ocean) or a fan on or turn on a radio on between stations. That brings in enough competing noise that is helps take your focus off the tinnitus. Or, I can lend you one of my more annoying relatives that will jaw at ya until the tinnitus is just a fading memory. (Just kidding, Aunt Eunice!!)

Why does tinnitus happen (that is not medically-related)?? Well, I'm glad you asked. I have a theory about that. It may be insane, but I believe it to be accurate. In essence, it is a knowledgeable compilation of several proven theories out there. But take it with a grain of salt and call it Tonya's Theory (aren't all theories named after the humble people who discovered them??).

Tonya's Tinnitus Origins Theory: In the inner ear are teeny weenie inner hair cells, or hairs. The duty of these hairs is to convey meaningful information from sounds that come into the ear by converting them into nerve impulses that are then sent to the brain to be interpreted. These hairs are in different places on the cochlea and give a pitch-specific sound when cued, like the keys of a piano. That part isn't my theory- all that is proven fact. Here it is now... sometimes when those hairs are damaged (either because of loud noise exposure or dehydration or ototoxicity- poison from some strong medications or agents- or environmental toxins or low blood flow or just genetics plus time, etc.), they weaken and break off and are dissolved, resulting in a hearing loss. Again, that part is proven. **Sometimes**, however, those hairs do **not** break off completely, but just stay bent or damaged, so that they are constantly giving the brain that pitch impulse. This is why only you hear that sound. The hairs think they are doing their job, but they are damaged... it's like a record that skips. That's it. Most people here say, "Oh that makes sense." And in my humble opinion, it makes sense to me too. There are a lot of other opinions out there, so bear that in mind.

The sound stays at the same volume all the time, but is only heard when sounds around you are not equal to the task of covering it up. A hearing aid helps in many cases where a hearing loss is present because it helps you to hear the sounds coming in around you loud enough and at the right pitches to dispel your focus away from the tinnitus. The tinnitus is still there... you just don't hear it anymore. Of course, it doesn't work for everyone... just like not everyone likes catsup on their scrambled eggs- yummy.

There are things that exacerbate/worsen the tinnitus, and I will touch briefly on those. Caffeine, alcohol (or other dehydrating agents), nicotine, stress, depression, certain medication or agents, loud noise/music/movie exposure, lack of physical fitness, and high salt diets will cause the tinnitus to worsen. The good news is that the worsening effect is usually temporary and returns to its prior state when you stop doing those things. So, it is to your advantage to live a healthy life, stay hydrated, and keep fit! Broken record, I know, and I realize I'm not your gym teacher or fitness trainer, but it really is true.

One more quick word before I leave this intriguing topic. Please do not go trying out every herbal remedy you see on the shelf or hear about on the internet!!! For one thing, most of them have been proven to be no better than a placebo (fake medicine), and for another, it can be very dangerous.

One herbal remedy, specifically gingko biloba, has been found to be effective around 25% of the time, but it is a blood thinner and must never be used in conjunction with other blood thinners, aspirine products, or certain blood pressure medications. B complex vitamins have also had some measure of success for some patients (about 25% of the time). If in doubt, either don't do it or ask your trusted physician or pharmacist first. Every other remedy out there that I know of is fake, a money-making scam, or nonsense... proven no better than a placebo. I'm sorry to have to tell you that, but I would rather you spend your money on that fabulous trip to Tahiti- it will relax you more also. Matter of fact, that sounds pretty good... see ya there!

Chapter 3
Audiologist vs. Hearing Instrument Specialist

When you need to have a heart operation, would you go to a guy who used to sell cars but took 6 months of on the job training and paid to pass a test and now operates on hearts? If you said yes, I cannot help you... no one can. If you said no, however, you have just agreed that it is better to take your important hearing needs to your Audiologist than a hearing instrument specialist/dealer/prosthetologist (my favorite)/salesperson. If you would only trust something as important as your heart to a cardiologist, a heart professional, it seems only right that you would only trust something as important as your hearing to an Audiologist, a hearing professional.

Sound a little extreme? Well, let's explore that a little. An Audiologist, to be certified and licensed, has to have a minimum of a Masters degree in Audiology in order to practice and have served 9 to 11 months full time under another Audiologist (called the clinical fellowship year, comparable to a physician's residency in their field of study). Now, all new Audiologists have to have a professional doctorate in Audiology, which is 4 years of additional education on top of their undergraduate degree, and 11 months clinical fellowship year. A hearing instrument specialist (or other titles) had 6 months (at most) of on the job training and passed a test about hearing aids. That is a marked difference in both education and ethics.

Wait, did she say ethics? At the risk of getting a whole lot of people angry with me (particularly hearing instrument specialists), yes, I said ethics.   Why? Well, I'm glad you asked. If you are selling hearing aids without knowing what you are doing, you are cutting corners and choosing to make money rather than seek to understand the best interest of the patient. If you are selling hearing aids because you tired of selling cars, how can you possibly have the best interest and understanding of the patient?

Don't get me wrong, there are some ethical dispensers out there... **some**. There are good and bad of every profession... good and bad physicians, good and bad Audiologists, good and bad salespeople, etc. However, even a bad Audiologist still understands the hearing system and when to refer for medical treatment and when to fit hearing aids.

Let me tell you some secret inside stuff, at the risk of ticking off a lot of people, but because I care about you and/or your loved ones. I have heard true and reliable stories from my patients that tell me about their experience with hearing instrument specialists. I have heard of them charging my patients the same amount or more for hearing aids that are not worth a tenth of the value they are selling them for, calling them the best on the market. Yet, they have fabulous full page ads in the paper!

For example, a patient the other day told me that he paid $4,200 for a set of Miracle Ear hearing aids (in this instance). I know for a fact that the dispenser was able to purchase them for around $220 each. And, the hearing aids were never satisfactory in performance to the patient... they didn't even have noise reduction or feedback cancellation (we'll go into that later)!! What's worse, when my patient read the small print about getting his money back (except for a deposit and restocking fee) within 30 days of purchase if not satisfied, he was instructed several times after adjustments to try for another week until the 30 days were over and it was too late to get his money back. This burns my butt! Do you think this is an isolated case??? I could go on and on with the stories my patients tell me. I won't, because I'm mad already, but I will tell you one more.

A new patient came in to my office the other day telling me that he was just to a hearing aid dispenser in town who fitted him with a hearing aid. He had me check it because it wasn't working. I called the manufacturer to see if it was still under warranty for repairs. The company told me it had been out of warranty since October of 2004. That means this hearing aid was purchased as stock by the dispenser in October of 2003 at the latest and was sold to him as great technology and new in 2008!!! I asked how much he had paid for this $130 hearing aid, and he told me $900.

These two stories are fresh in my mind because they are the latest ones I heard, not because they are the worst (believe me!) or the only ones. So, I would not only recommend going to an Audiologist, but I would also check with the Better Business Bureau before you go anywhere. And trust me, if there is a full page ad that promises a very inexpensive hearing aid... do remember that it may very well be a sales trap. They may say that the inexpensive lure won't work for you or say it's only if you buy one at the manufacturer's retail price (which is always about double what you'd pay normally). You **always** get what you pay for.

So, you ask, how do I know the difference? How do I avoid this terrible fate? How do I keep from being swindled? Help me! Okay, calm down... I got your back. Here is how you know the difference. Are you ready for this one? Now, prepare yourself... ask. Before you make an appointment, you call them up and say, "Would I be seeing an Audiologist?" If you don't want to be so direct, you can take a peek at the letters after their name. If they are an Audiologist, they will have either "M.S., CCC-A" or "M.S., FAAA" or "M.A., CCC-A" or "M.A., FAAA". That means a Masters of Science or Art and a clinical certificate of competence in Audiology through the American Speech-Language and Hearing Association (CCC-A) or a fellow of the American Audiology Association (FAAA). It's that simple. If they don't have those letters or have a H.I.S. (hearing instrument specialist) or something like that, they are not Audiologists but hearing instrument specialists.

Trust your hearing health to a hearing professional, for your sake as well as ours. Plus, I'm getting sick of the stories... come to me first and you won't have to buy two sets (because you absolutely hate the first set or were fitted wrong)! You really could go to Tahiti!!!

Chapter 4
How Did This Happen? or Why Me?

Why would something like a hearing loss happen? Well, it's probably because of something bad you've done. Or maybe you are a very bad person and are being paid back for it. Or maybe you went to a loud concert as a teenager. Or perhaps you didn't walk your dog when you were twelve and you lied about it to your parents. I hope you're catching my drift that these are really silly reasons and probably don't contribute much to your hearing loss, and yet many of my patients think some very strange things and even had a great deal of guilt along with. Please don't put yourself through more stress than you already are under and read on.

Before I get into the possible etiologies/causes, let me start by reminding you that hearing losses can afflict themselves on anyone, even children, who have done nothing wrong but maybe take a little too much time to potty train. It is vital for you to not beat yourself up about it. Most people want to know why, but knowing does nothing to change the current situation, and the treatment will be the same.

Some hearing losses occur because of excessive noise exposure. It usually is repeated noise bombardment from work or lots of time with a fun hobby, like woodworking, band playing, Harley riding, or power tool use, etc. Or, hunters pay attention here, from a single rifle or pistol shot or many. Then again, of course, servicemen and women can have too much noise exposure in their jobs that may not be able to be prevented in war times. And let me take this time to thank you for your service to our country! My dad was a Marine, and I appreciate your service so much that allows us to have peace and freedom in our great land!!!

Of course, some people are exposed to the same amount of noise as you and never drop their hearing a single decibel (at least until much later than you). That has to do with genetic predispositions. Those people whose passion it is to do nothing but research all their lives have discovered more genetic involvement in hearing loss than previously thought. Apart from noise exposure, some people exhibit hearing loss who have never heard an amplified rock concert or even mowed a lawn.

Apart from genetics and noise exposure, there are other contributing factors or causes that are less common. Ototoxicity (harmful effects to the ears by medications) can occur with strong (intravenous) antibiotics, chemotherapeutic drugs, and some other strong medications (usually life-saving). Very high fevers (usually over 104 degrees) can cause damage, especially if they are sustained. Dehydration (generally sustained or severe or related to alcoholism) can cause fluid levels in the inner ear to be reduced and cause hair cells to dry out, which may cause damage. Toxicity by nicotine occurs in the ears as well as the rest of the body, causing temporary to permanent hearing loss (as well as will accentuating tinnitus/ringing), depending on the duration and genetics of the patient. A car accident or beating sometimes will cause a permanent hearing loss (or could be temporary), depending on the severity and recovery process. Sometimes, for children especially, permanent hearing loss happens in the womb if the mommy has a high fever or other illness during certain months of development (German measles is a big player).

Some hearing losses are permanent that involve only the middle part of the ear because the patient is not a surgical candidate or chooses not to undergo surgery. It is also possible that the surgery for the middle ear only restored a portion of the hearing or none at all (in some rare cases), and further help is necessary. These middle ear conditions may be from the ossicles (those three tiny bones in the middle ear- the smallest bones in your body) discontinuity, burst eardrum (although that's rare- it usually heals itself or can be surgically replaced easily), or otosclerosis (the fusing/calcifying of the bones).

The most annoying thing is when nothing causes it... it just happens. This is the hardest for people to accept. We want to blame someone, something. It is a hard pill to swallow to just be dealt a poor hand. Well, I am a firm believer that everything happens for a reason. Even if it's horrid, we can grow from it, deepen our understanding of others' pain, help others going through the same thing for the first time, or even just help others grow by allowing them to help you sometimes.

So, for whatever reason listed above, you or your loved one has the hearing loss. Again, I want to emphasize that moving forward is the best course of action, not dwelling on why it happened to you. Dwelling on why keeps you in the past, a poor victim, while dwelling on moving forward keeps you in the present, an intelligent overcomer. ☺

Chapter 5
Getting There From Here and Ear Stuff

The funniest thing I ever heard someone say was, "You can't get there from here." It's usually when giving directions and is then followed by how you **can** get there, normally instructions to go back to such and such a highway, road, etc. and then go such and such a way. It still gives me a chuckle.

Fortunately with a permanent hearing loss, you can get to better hearing from here. There is a way to hear again, understand again, be part of the conversation again, enjoy the TV and movies again, etc. After it's discovered that the treatment is not medication or surgery, the only medical treatment that will work is tiny little devices called hearing aids.

One option of hearing aids, for those with severe to profound hearing losses, is a surgically-implanted hearing aid. There are two main types... a bone-anchored hearing aid (for those with chronic middle ear problems) and an inner ear/cochlear implant. These can be implanted on one or both sides, depending on the situation. For these, you have to have a certain severity of hearing loss and meet a list of additional criteria as well. Many insurance companies reimburse for the procedures and follow-ups but many also do not. (Your insurance company can be called to check eligibility and benefits if you qualify for an implant.)

These surgically-implanted hearing aids are very good options for people who fit into the criteria, especially those who have very poor discrimination/word understanding, leaving them un-helped by traditional hearing aids. Remember that they are permanent. You can't go back to traditional forms of hearing aids afterwards in most cases (all cases of cochlear implants that I know of). If you are interested, there are tons of websites available or books, if computers aren't your thing. The three companies at this time that manufacture implants in no order are Med-El (an Austrian company), Advanced Bionics (an American company), and Cochlear Corporation (an Australian company, I think). Another option I would recommend is to see an Audiologist or Otorhinolaryngologist (who comes up with these names??)/Ear, Nose, and Throat (ENT) Physician, and they will tell you if you would be a good candidate or not and refer you accordingly.

The most common forms of hearing aids, however, by far are traditional hearing aids, those devices that are worn in or on/behind the ear, fitted (hopefully) by Audiologists. These are widely worn and utilized by intelligent people who have decided to participate in the conversation despite their hearing difficulties.

What is a hearing aid exactly? Well, am I so glad you asked me. In its most basic (and unpleasant) form, it is simply a microphone (to pick up the sound), amplifier (to make the sound louder), and a receiver (to deliver the amplified sound back to you). That is basically all the older analog hearing aids were. That is what the cheapies are still ($19.95 per personal one-size-fits-all amplifier I've seen in magazines).

What a hearing aid is not is just as important. A hearing aid is not a normal ear... never will be. I know that seems funny, but believe me there are people who believe that a hearing aid should be just as good as a normal ear. If anyone ever tells you that will happen, they lie. It will not give you bionic hearing or hear what is said two or twelve rooms away or whisper the time or news in your ear on demand (however, that's a good idea) or turn off at will in the presence of annoying talkers, etc.

So, let's talk about the steps leading up to the determination of wearing hearing aids and what your expectations should be. By now, you've probably had a comprehensive audiometric/hearing evaluation. I've mentioned it but not described it, so let's do that for those interested. If you're not one of those interested, feel free to skip down to the paragraph that begins, "All righty then."

A hearing examination should minimally include the following elements... a very thorough hearing history, with questions about past testing/results, lifestyle, family history, and previous aid use if applicable. Then, you should have an otoscopic evaluation (the little light and magnifying glass thing) to check out the outer ear up to the eardrum/tympanic membrane.

Once that is complete, the rest of the evaluation should occur in a sound-treated booth. (If no booth is present, run away... run far, run fast- huge clue to their attention to accuracy of testing.) So, once seated in the booth, headphones are put on/in and a tight squeezing band put onto the bone behind the ear on one side and in front of the ear on the other side. You may be given a push button for your responses or be instructed to raise your hand. (Again, if they don't put a bone conduction headband on you, run, because they only want to put a hearing aid on you even if the loss is medically treatable.)

So, you'll then be instructed to push the button or raise your hand each and every time you hear a little beep. This is for air conduction testing, to evaluate the entire ear system (outer ear, middle ear, inner ear, and some parts of the brain. We are looking for the softest sound you can here for this, so respond even if you barely hear it. This beep can and should change pitch, sometimes be a high tone and sometimes a low tone and everywhere in between.

Why are beeps used? Well, am I glad you asked! We want to test the individual frequencies/pitches of speech, because those are the most meaningful sounds we hear every day. Beeps rather than speech are used to isolate different pitch/frequency information. Speech changes pitch like crazy naturally. There can be low and high frequency/pitch information in one word. Think of it, for example, in the word "note"... the "no" part of that word is low pitched, but the "te" part at the end is high pitched. And there are millions of other examples (well at least thousands). So, if we used only speech information, the hearing loss would be very general and not specific enough to yield enough information to program a hearing aid to give you what you need specifically.

Okay, so that process is performed for each ear individually (again for specificity). And if you liked that, good, because that entire thing will be repeated **again** for the bone conduction part of it. Bone conduction tesing bypasses the ear canal, ear drum, and middle ear to tell us directly what the inner ear is doing. Often times, masking (the addition of wind/static noise to the ear opposite to the one we are testing to rule out its involvement) is required to obtain correct responses. Sometimes masking is not needed if bone conduction results match the air conduction results.

So, that fun is over now, it is time to move on to speech testing, and words are used from here on out rather than beeps. The first speech test we do is called Speech Recognition Threshold testing, and it is to determine to softest word you can understand enough to repeat. So, we will say silly words like "bathtub, railroad, rainbow," etc. and ask you to say them back to us. Its purpose is to verify the air conduction testing and see if there are discrepancies, which could mean either there is a problem we need to explore or you're a faker (which is a little more common in children).

We Audiologists are a touch evil here on purpose in that we drop the words down to where you can no longer repeat them and then come back up to where you can again. The evil part is people think for a moment or two that their hearing problem is worse than they thought or the family member listening is a little freaked out, and some even get frustrated or panicky just for a second. The reason we are evil like that is to verify our results and that's it.

The last speech test we must perform is Word Recognition Scores testing. During this test, the Audiologist will say some sentences like, "Say the word cat." The patient's job is to say the word "cat" at the end of the sentence. Please don't repeat the entire sentence, as we hear it enough as it is and are only interested in the last word.

This test seems silly, but it serves a very important purpose... it shows us how well the nerve and brain are functioning with regard to your understanding ability. This is a quick scan also for certain serious medical problems that can arise in the system, such as acoustic neuromas (tumors) or damaged/severed/pinched nerves, etc. For instance, last month, in my office, I referred two different patients to an ear, nose, and throat physician, who scheduled an MRI for them, which showed acoustic neuromas/tumors for each of them. Don't worry... they were treated surgically and are fine now, and they are really not all that common. How did I suspect this? Well, the hearing was asymmetric (different for each ear), and that loss was accompanied by very different word recognition scores in each ear. So, silly or not it's important, so humor us.

Another optional test is to determine most comfortable listening levels and uncomfortable listening levels. It is my opinion that this is important to do before fitting hearing aids, for instance, or to determine if a person is very/too sensitive to loud noises (something called hyperacousis). What does that matter? Well, I'll talk about why a little later when I discuss how hearing aids work.

Most comfortable and uncomfortable listening level testing is performed using either words or beeps. I prefer words, because it is more real-life, but everyone is different. For most comfortable listening level testing, running words or a series of beeps are presented, and the patient is asked either for their level of comfort with the presentation of the beeps or their comfort in listening to words at that level for an extended period of time. For uncomfortable loudness levels, the person is presented with increasingly loud stimulus and asked to respond when to the point of insanity. Not really, but that would be interesting (insert evil laugh). Rather, the patient is asked to respond when the sound/words are too loud, "as in you wouldn't want to hear something that loud for more than a couple seconds". Again, not every Audiologist performs these two tests, but I feel it is valuable information.

So, there is the normal test battery in a comprehensive Audiometric examination/evaluation. It normally includes otoscopy (looking in the ear), air conduction testing, bone conduction testing, and speech audiometric testing (speech reception thresholds and word recognition scores testing). That is the normal gamut of testing. Any extras are just that... extra. This may or may not be beneficial information but will definitely cost extra.

Some Audiologists also throw in tympanometry, which puts a little plug in your ear and a little pressure in and back out against your eardrum to test the eardrum's compliance, middle ear pressure, and ear canal volume. This is important information with a conductive hearing loss or mixed hearing loss, which we will discuss in a moment or two. With children, this test is valuable, as the majority of hearing losses in children occur with middle ear involvement.

Some Audiologists will perform otoacoustic emissions (OAE) testing. This test is just holding still and listening to tones for a little bit... no response is necessary. It is a sweet little test that shows us the outer hair cell function. Again, I'll talk about that soon. It is a nice objective test when people can't respond that well for whatever reason.

Some Audiologists also regularly screen for acoustic neuromas (tumors of the hearing system) with either a tone decay test or acoustic reflexes and decay testing. The tone decay test is the presentation of a long beep, and the patient is asked to tell the Audiologist when the sound goes away. Acoustic reflexes and decay are less gentle and present loud beeps to see how the muscles and nerves are working together to elicit a stapedial muscle contraction or "startle" response to loud sounds.

These tests can be helpful if the patient history indicates it as a possibility. They are not normally done, however, due to time constraints and large price tags of the equipment for some of these tests.

All righty then. There are many other tests that Audiologists can perform and interpret, but those mentioned are the ones related to strictly hearing testing in terms of evaluating for hearing aids. I hope that information was useful.

So, what does the test/audiogram show us? I'm glad you asked. The hearing test is a reflection of how well you are hearing **and** understanding (which are two very different things). It is a reflection of what is going on in the entire ear system from the outer ear (cartilage to the eardrum), middle ear (those tiny little bones to the oval window), inner ear (cochlea- outer and inner hair cells, etc.), and cranial nerves (cranial nerve VIII and cranial nerve VII for the stapedial reflex) to the cortex for interpretation and response.

The audiogram tells us how well you are hearing through the entire ear system (air conduction testing) and the inner ear alone (bone conduction testing) and can give us an idea of your understanding. The word recognition testing provides information about the understanding of speech when the sound is loud enough. For example, missing zero to two words out of 25 is considered an excellent neural response, missing three to five words is considered good, missing six to seven words is considered fair, and missing eight or more is considered poor.

So, with the test results, the Audiologist can determine how to treat your particular hearing problem. If it is conductive (having to do with something going on in the outer or middle part of your ear), the Audiologist will refer you to your primary care physician or ear, nose, and throat specialist physician, etc. Some people these days are opting for the slightly less expensive alternatives, such as a nurse practitioner or physician's assistant as the first healthcare professionals they go to for conductive hearing losses. Other people want to go straight to the physician ear specialist. Everyone is different, and much will depend upon your insurance coverage or lack thereof.

A conductive loss may simply require a dosage of antibiotic (if it's an infection), either oral or ear drops or both, or an allergy test or drying agent (if it's likely allergy or sinus related), or be as complex as a surgical consultation (if the middle ear bones are disconnected or calcified or eardrum is perforated). This type of hearing loss is treatable.

A mixed type of hearing loss has parts that are conductive and parts that are sensorineural (which we talk about in the next paragraph).

For this type of loss, the conductive hearing loss should be treated and then the patient re-evaluated to see how much the hearing improves before treatment for a sensorineural hearing loss ensues.

A sensorineural hearing loss is what we're going to park on. This type of hearing loss is a permanent type of hearing loss. It used to be called "nerve deafness", but that is a gross representation most of the time. I still see patients regularly who had their physicians tell them forty years ago that nothing could be done. I believe at the time they were also bleeding patients of their bad blood to "cure them" of illnesses. Whereas that may have been the case way back when, or at least the limited knowledge or technology we possessed, we are now living with the miraculous power of technology... oohhhh... aaahhhh. Even those who do have true nerve deafness, as in are deaf (hearing thresholds equal to or worse than 85 decibels hearing level) and have very poor word recognition scores are possibly candidates of cochlear implants.

Speaking of degrees of hearing loss... let's, shall we? With any type of hearing loss, there are varying degrees of severity. It's very similar to vision in that way. There are people who only have minor problems with clarity of vision and some that can't see the broad side of a barn and everything in between. With hearing there are slight or mild losses that may only decrease the volume or acuity of hearing a little or people that can't hear the broad side of a barn. Okay, so not the best analogy, but you know what I mean, I think. Well, the severity is the same with all types of hearing losses (conductive, mixed, or sensorineural), I will be focusing the rest of our little one-sided discussion (actually, you are welcome to talk back to the pages, I just can't hear you) on sensorineural hearing losses, which is what I treat.

An audiogram is a graph of where the hearing level thresholds are at various pitches. The shape of this and its values determine the severity of the hearing loss. An example is below, in Figure 1. You read it that the vertical lines represent the different pitches, ranging from low pitch on the left to high pitch on the right. The horizontal lines represent how loud that particular pitched sound has to be to hear it, so it is the loudness in decibels of hearing level. The further down your hearing is plotted on the chart, the worse your hearing is.

A slight hearing loss is a term generally restricted for use with kids who are still developing language and learning their reading, writing, and 'rithmetic. A slight hearing loss can affect early learning very negatively and is generally worse (in my opinion) because most people don't opt or aren't able to do anything about it, so it remains untreated. I say it is worse because a slight or mild hearing loss untreated is worse than a more severe hearing loss that is treated (as long as it is treated right).

I won't bore you with all the categories, because they are easier to understand by reading the paragraph above the audiogram picture and looking at the shading areas. The audiogram is showing a slight to moderately-severe hearing loss. The results were from the right ear, as they have circles on the intersection of the vertical and horizontal lines. Left ear is represented by an "X". So when you see "X"'s and "O"'s, it doesn't mean kisses and hugs, but it means left ear and right ear... nice try.

Figure 1: Audiogram

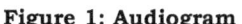

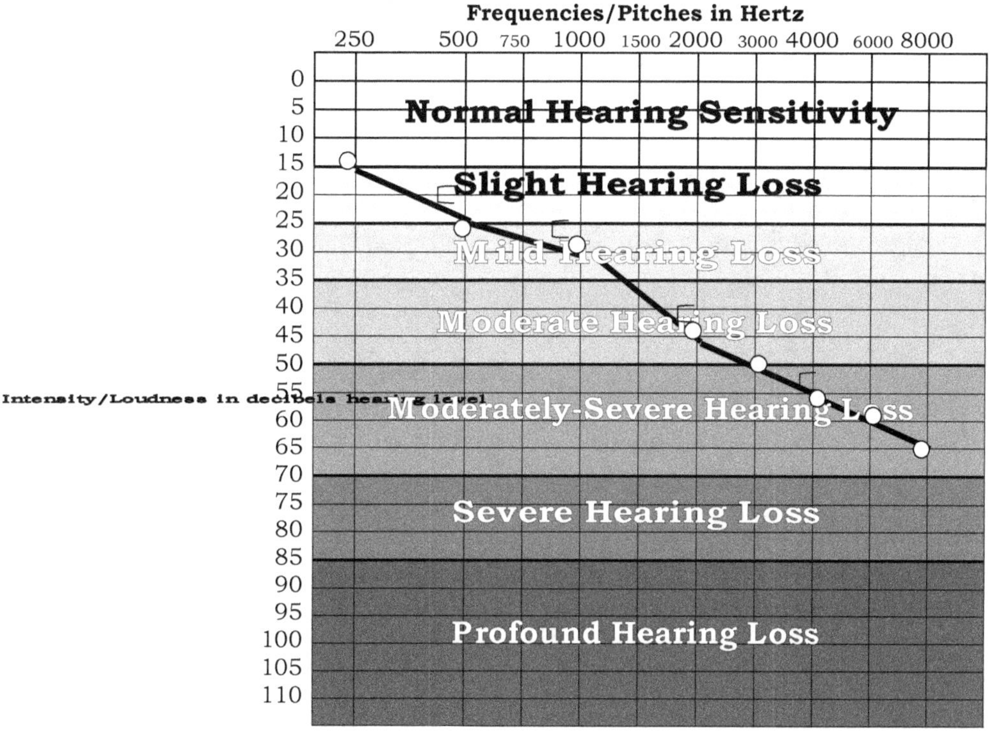

Bone conduction scores are represented by the symbol "<" for right ear and ">" for the left ear, but masked results are represented by "[" for the right and "]" for the left.

Bone conduction directly stimulates the inner ear, whereas air conduction stimulates the entire ear system (outer, middle, and inner ear). If there is a discrepancy between the two, it is considered a conductive or mixed hearing loss, depending on whether those bone conduction scores fall within normal limits (the former) or reveal a hearing loss (the latter). That is when the tester should refer to your physician or ENT (ear, nose, and throat) physician specialist for further evaluation.

If the bone and air conduction scores are the same, there is no middle or outer ear problem that is severe enough to show up on an audiogram... or it is not bad enough to reveal itself as a hearing loss. If you are symptomatic for middle ear problems, like having pain in the ears, tinnitus/ringing in the ears all of a sudden, etc., it is still a good idea to see a physician or physician's assistant to nip any potential problems in the bud.

Okay, so we should move on to what to do with all this information. Let's assume your loving Audiologist has discovered a sensorineural (inner ear), permanent hearing loss. If it is mild or slight and you are an adult, it is a personal preference whether you pursue amplification. Some Audiologists recommend utilizing hearing assistive devices/aids with a mild hearing loss, because some conversations will be affected negatively with a mild hearing loss, especially in the presence of background noise/talking/music/etc.

Personally, I recommend this if the patient is still working and his/her job is dependent on understanding people. I also recommend it if the patient is very social and is being hindered from social activities and is starting to withdraw out of embarrassment or awkwardness (if that is a word) or frustration because of mishearing people. Also, there are some people that truly need hearing aids because they tell me they do. I think people know when they need hearing aids because they know themselves better than anyone (though I will never aid a patient without some hearing loss present).

For most people, however, hearing aids will be recommended certainly for anyone in the moderate hearing loss range or worse. This is the group I will address for the remainder of the book. I will do my best to answer some of the important questions most people have and inform you of what is truth and what are lies.

Chapter 6
Why are they so expensive?

Anyone who says hearing aids are cheap are either delusional or have way too much money and should share with the rest of the class. There are a lot of gimmicks out there (the most popular is two for the price of one- at the manufacturer's retail price, that is, which just happens to be double the normal price after all). But in my experience, you get what you pay for. Sometimes there are great sales on hearing aids, but you discover after testing that those conveniently won't work for you (the old bait and switch is still alive today, though more cleverly disguised). So, in my humble opinion, stay away from the gimmicks. In my office, I have one price for each level of technology (very basic, enhanced basic, midline, and top-of-the-line). As of 2008, my prices range from $1,000 to $2,600 each, depending on which level of technology you need/want/can afford. There are very little price differences in different sizes of hearing aids, so I don't change my price for different sizes (completely-in-the-canals to behind-the-ears, etc.).

The old hearing aids, meaning the ones made before about 2000-2001, were all analog hearing aids. What does that mean? Well, it means that the ingredients inside the hearing aid were: a microphone, a basic amplifier, a receiver, and the casing. If you were lucky, you got potentiometers that could manually adjust the high pitches, low pitches, overall gain, etc. If you had a really good "modern" one, it could be programmed on the computer, but the ingredients in the aids were the same. Some amplifiers were better or stronger than others, but the circuit was decided by your audiogram at the moment of testing.

So, why don't we have these available anymore? Well, they are available from some manufacturers, but the cost is not that much less than the least expensive digital hearing aids these days. In addition, you get what you pay for.

It is not in your best interest to buy analog hearing aids new. Along with the cursory ingredients in them, the downsides to them are as follows: squealing/whistling/feedback when you have them loud enough to hear, no noise reduction so noise is as loud or louder than speech, wind blowing over the microphone is bothersome, chewing is heard above anything else, everything is amplified evenly despite what you really need (for the most part), sound like an 8-track tape (if you're old enough to remember what that sounds like), and that's about all I can think of off hand. These are the problems people have had for years before **good** digital aids (not just the **first** digital aids) came out. That is why many people bought them and threw them in a drawer. And if you do that, any price is too high.

The programmable analog hearing aids were very similar in problems but got a little closer to matching the hearing aid with the targets of the audiogram. They were much better, but still had all the downsides of feedback, noise, and others. And a lot of less-than-honest, let's say, dispensers and even Audiologists (sorry to say) called them digital because they had a computer chip in them, but they were only programming an analog circuit not digitally processing the sound.

Enter Resound on the scene, the first manufacturer of digital sound processing inside digital hearing aids and still the leader in hearing aid technology in the world. Yes, many other manufacturers claim to be **and many are** very good, but these guys are the real deal and are my unabashed preference. (My second favorite is Phonak.) But let me say, there are many good leaders in technology of hearing aids these days that are very good too, such as Widex, Siemens, Starkey's Destiny line, Unitron, Rexton, etc. Let me say again that Resound is **my** personal favorite... not that any other ones are necessarily bad- they aren't. Everyone has their own favorite company. Anyway, the first ones didn't have noise reduction inside them, but they did have a sound more like a CD- clearer- and better volume without the feedback. The best thing about the early digital hearing aids is that you could program it to give volume pretty much where you needed it **only**. That was huge!

Along the years, technology improvements eventually crept into the hearing aids, and now they are better than they have ever been. They are still not perfect, but nothing is ever going to exactly duplicate all the intricate workings and amazing sound of originally normal hearing. Why? Because there is no better designed or functioning computer in the world than the human brain!! Hands down, they will never ever **ever** be able to duplicate it... believe me they have tried and will continue to do so. That doesn't keep us from expecting it to, but that's another matter.

Our natural hearing system is extraordinarily complex. Digital programming and processing and digital filters for noise and feedback (that obnoxious whistling noise that happens when hearing aids are completely covered up or not fit properly) are manufactured to perform great feats in a very small compartment.

The hearing aids now are miniature computers, capable of many, but not all, of the natural hearing processes up to the level of the hearing nerve. From then on it becomes the brain's responsibility to transmit the proper information via the hearing nerve to the temporal brain lobe (mostly), assign meaning to that information, interpret and process it, and then decide if some action is required of other parts of the brain/body. All this is done in micro or milliseconds (as long as no parts of that system are weakened). It's quite amazing!

For instance, a sound produces sound waves in the air that come in through the ear canal to stimulate the eardrum, which causes eardrum vibrations whose intensity of vibration parallels the intensity of sound. That vibration of the eardrum causes mechanical movement of the three tiniest bones in your body, located in the middle ear. Remember the hammer (malleus), anvil (incus), and stirrup (stapes)? Yeah, those. So, the mechanical movement, like a pumping action that's intensity parallels the intensity of vibration from the eardrum, pushes and pulls on a little oval window or door the stapes/stirrup is attached to. This movement transfers mechanical energy to hydraulic energy, as the space on the other side of the window/door is filled with fluid. Very simply speaking, the pushing/pulling of the door produces little waves that crash on the shore (basilar membrane) where tiny little hairs (hair cells) live. Again, how hard the waves crash on the delicate little hairy shore depends on how hard the window/door is pushed and pulled, which parallels how hard the bones are pumping and how much vibration the eardrum elicits. Well, these little hairs that are embedded on the shore (simply speaking) are pitch/frequency-specific. They are laid out on the shore in tonal order, going from high pitch on down the shore to low pitch. Because this would take too much room to lay it straight, it is curled up into a shape like a snail shell, which is why it is called the cochlea, which is Latin for snail-shaped. Ironic, isn't it? So, high pitch information produces shorter-soundwave vibrations in the eardrum and equal movements in the bones of the middle ear and tiny pushes and pulls on the window/door and waves that hit the hairy shore close to the door in the high pitch area. The area is very frequency-pitch specific. How hard it does all this depends on the loudness of the sound, and the harder the waves hit, the more hairs are stimulated so they add up to more/louder sound detected. Well, then those little hairs, when moved/stimulated by the crashing wave, produces a tiny electrical charge that travels quickly to the hearing/acoustic nerve it is connected to. So, the hydraulic energy becomes electrical energy. Then, the electrical charge travels from the hearing nerve to the cortex of the brain in the temporal lobe region (mostly) for sound processing and interpretation. Then, depending on what the sound is interpreted as being, more nerves fire to the locations of the brain that need to respond.

For instance, a loud siren is heard and interpreted as a loud siren. Things closer to us are louder than things farther away, so we can tell if it is moving toward us of not. Also, our brain processes information from both of our ears simultaneously, so that it can determine which ear (if any) is receiving louder information, indicating that the sound is closer to one ear than the other. That is how we localize or determine where sound occurs in relation to our body. So, we can tell where the sound is, how loud it is, whether it's moving closer to us or farther away, and signals the legs to move to get out of the way if necessary.

If words come into the ear, the brain interprets them and responds as appropriate with action of the body or a word response or both. Again, all this complexity is performed within micro or milliseconds, depending on the age and other factors of the person. It is very remarkable!

As you may have deduced, the brain actually does most of the work of interpreting and the ears do most of the work of giving the brain the correct information as much as it is capable of. The danger of loud noises is that the incoming waves crash on those delicate little hairs so hard that some of them can be damaged or uprooted. We have millions of them, so it takes some repetition and time for the effects of it to be seen on a hearing test. In fact, the best estimate is that 40% of those hairs are toast before any hearing loss shows up on a hearing test. The scary part of that is that a lot of damage has already been done before you see any effects of it. This damage can occur at any age. There are genetic predispositions to hearing loss also, so some people are more affected by noise damage than others.

Generally, for those exposed to loud or repeatedly loud noises throughout life or even long ago, a hearing loss begins in the high pitches. The reason is that the hairs for the high pitches are closest to that window/door. And let me take this moment to tell you that damaging noise can come from machinery, saws, airplane jets, gunshots, ipods, MP3 players, tractors, drills, baby cries, musical instruments, speakers, truck noise, industrial fans, motors, vacuums, lawn mowers, leaf blowers, etc. To prevent a hearing loss and especially when a hearing loss is already determined, it is vital to protect your ears from further damage by wearing earplugs/hearing protection around loud noises to keep it from worsening quickly.

I got off track a little bit, but I wanted to go into some detail about the normal hearing process to make this point... a hearing aid has to try to do all that the ear does up to the hairy shore level in a tiny electronic and digital device. People expect a hearing aid to make their hearing as good as their normal ear, but it never will. Even the best aids on the market are still aids, not ears. They are better than they've ever been, but our expectations are much higher than they've ever been also. The nerves and brain are still the ones responsible primarily for interpreting sound, determining where sound is located, separating noise from meaningful sounds or speech, yielding understanding from what is heard, and so on. The hearing aids just help get the sounds to the brain for interpretation. Does that make sense?

So, why are they so expensive? Well, the cost of living has gone up, technology is better than ever before, hearing aid manufacturers are in the business of making money and have to pay a lot for marketing, hearing aid dispensers are in the business of making money, Audiologists have to live and need to make money, marketing is expensive, inflation happens, taxes are killing us, gas prices are enormous, and there are a high quantity of American alligators now in Florida again. Okay, that last one isn't so relevant, but I'm sure a dollar or two goes into some kind of environment protection somewhere. In short, they just are. I wish they weren't- really, it would make my job easier and allow more people to have them that need them- but they are.

What is a reasonable price for a good hearing aid? It ranges, depending on the amount of technology you need (specifically how much noise you are around on a regular basis). In my office, it ranges from $1,000 to $2,600 each. Many others are more and some are less. In general, you get what you pay for, but that being said, regardless of the technology, **if you pay more than $5,900 or $6,000, you are being taken for a ride!** That is my informed opinion. I'll probably get a lot of angry calls about that, but it is the truth, so bring it on. I'm over people being taken advantage of, especially when in reality we are all on a "fixed income" these days.

This is good stuff, isn't it? Are we learning a lot? I hope so. Let's continue with a look at the differences between hearing aids.

Chapter 7
A Pinto verses a Cadillac

So, how much technology do you really need, anyway? Even more than that, what brand is really the best to invest in when everyone claims to be the best? Well, let me tell you.

The answer to that first technology question depends entirely on your hearing loss and your lifestyle. Our body's requirements in every way vary with the environments we are consistently in. If you are a businessman, still working, with meetings and conversations over dinner, and parties to attend, and your job performance requires that you understand people correctly, I would **definitely** aim for the highest technology you can afford.

Also, if you find yourself being very active socially or in the wind frequently (as in with golfing or fishing regularly) or dancing regularly or eating at restaurants more than twice a week, stick with the highest technology you can afford.

If, however, you mostly stay at home, watching TV, talking on the telephone, eat out once or twice a month, and just have quiet conversations with one or two people at a time, you really wouldn't be utilizing all that technology even if you had it, so it is a personal preference for you. You would probably be fine with saving yourself some money and stick with a more basic model.

You know yourself. If you are an engineer by trade and are very exacting and attuned to your environment and have very high demands on everyone, especially when technology or a lot of money are involved (yeah, you know who you are), well, please do your Audiologist a favor and go with the best technology. You know you want it to sound the best anyway… come on, you know it. A personal note here… engineers are my favorite clients (no offense, everyone else) because we get to know each other so well. They are in my office more than anyone else, trying to get it "just right". I love it! It is a very welcome challenge, and I enjoy it immensely.

If you are a more generally light-hearted and promotional in nature and whimsy and just as happy as a little bug to actively converse with people and socialize your life away, a more midline or top of the line technology would work for you, if you can afford it, depending on how often you go out. I steer you toward the better technology because what people say and interacting socially so very important to you. Heck, it's what you live for! I also love these patients, because they have great stories!

People in general who go out of their way to please everyone and keep the peace and are just as happy watching everyone enjoy themselves as actively participating, basic or midline generally is fine, depending on your lifestyle. Actually, if you fit into this category, you sweet thing, you probably made sure everyone else in the family's needs were met first and put it off until other people were complaining about your hearing loss. Even though you may not complain in general, and would tolerate a basic hearing aid, still get one that meets your needs. If you have a more active lifestyle, it is still important to be able to hear, and you just may need a midline hearing aid. Get what you need. For all that you do for others, don't deny yourself good hearing because of thinking you'd make do with less to allow those you love more. It's good for their sanity that you hear well. And please communicate your needs to your Audiologist so they can help. It's what we do. (Oh, and you particularly, please stay away from hearing aid dispensers because they may bully you, and that is not a healthy professional relationship.)

And for those large and in charge, you'll **tell** us what you need, so you just get what you want. That's all you're going to do anyway. I'm okay with that... just listen to the options first... humor me!

Okay, so definitely it is important to consider your personality and lifestyle when choosing the technology. How exactly does the technology differ? What difference does it make which technology you get?

For that answer, let me use the analogy of automobiles. All automobiles will get you from one place to another, but some will do so more comfortably than others.

A Pinto (sorry Pinto makers) is like a basic hearing aid... gets you there but your brain rattles a bit more in the process. It fills a need of hearing volume but not much else. This is the bare bones basic aid that is still digital and amplifies, but that's about it. The good news is that it is the most affordable technology (ranging from $900-$1,100 each); the bad news is that it amplifies everything equally- even things you may not want amplified. Also, for some manufacturers, it may squeal/ring/feed back on you. However, a basic hearing aid sometimes is all circumstance allows, and it is definitely better than no hearing aids at all. These generally come with a 1 year loss & damage and 1 year repair and remake warranty. The down side is no noise reduction, no feedback reduction filter, a less natural sound, one or two listening program(s) only and a phone program, and not as many color options for behind the ear hearing aids (I'll get into that later).

The next technology up is what I call the enhanced basic or value hearing aid, analogous to a Hyundai Accent ride- a little noisy and bumpy, but not as bad as a Pinto. (The Hyundai Accent was my first new car ever, and I liked the spunky little thing- and so reliable!) This digital aid includes some filters, though subtle/mild ones, that help filter out some unwanted sounds and should (these days) include a filter to help cancel and prevent feedback. This hearing aid, again, in my informed opinion, should be in the $1,500-$1,800 range each. It does a little more for you in noisy environments, but only helps a little with it. There are usually limitations, such as only 2 programs and the telecoil, fewer channels and bands (I'll get into that later), fewer programming options (for many manufacturers), a less natural sound than the better technologies, and a shorter warranty (generally 1 year loss & damage and 1 year repairs and remakes) than the higher technology aids.

The next technology up is the midline hearing aid. I would call this ride like a new Chevy Impala, with a little smoother and a little quieter ride. This digital aid includes a better filter to cancel out more noise, the feedback reduction/prevention filter, more channels, more program options (generally 3 programs and a telecoil program), more programming options, a more natural sound, and a longer warranty (generally 2 years loss & damage and repair and remake warranty). This aid is generally in the price range of $1,800-2,200 each, and again, that is my informed opinion.

The "top of the line" technology is the Cadillac of technology. It's a smooth, quiet (never silent) ride, with other little luxuries to make it more enjoyable. It has added wind noise reduction, reverberation reduction, more channels, more bands, the best noise filter, the feedback reduction/prevention filter, more natural sound, less noisy sound, walks and talks for you (okay, that one isn't true), longer warranty (generally 3 years loss & damage and repair and remake warranty). This aid should generally be in the price range of $2,500-$3,000 each. In my humble opinion, any more than that, you should go elsewhere, because you are being taken for an expensive ride.

Now, before I get onto my favorite hearing aid manufacturers and the actual best from the self-acclaimed best, let's get into what some of this high fangled technology talk really means to you. First, let's hit the channels and bands, because it is thrown around like popcorn popping as immense selling points, and sometimes unjustifiably so.

Let's start with what the word "channel" means with regards to hearing aids. However many channels the hearing aid has is how frequency-specific the aid can get or how well it will match your exact needs as it changes at different pitches. Now, remember the long discussion we had about how to interpret your hearing test/audiogram? It's still there, so you can go on back and re-read that if you need to. It's okay... I'll wait here for you if you need to review.

If you need 10 decibels (dB) of amplification/gain to reduce your hearing loss (or improve your hearing until it is close to normal) at 500 Hertz (Hz), a low pitch, but need 30 dB of amplification/gain to correct your hearing loss at 2,000 Hz, a high pitch, and had only 1 channel or sections of pitch to amplify, it would give you 20 dB amplification at both pitches. This would be annoying to listen to because you would be over-amplifying the low pitch and under-amplifying the high pitch, creating a noisy/loud environment without the clarity you need in understanding. This is why it is that in the olden days, hearing aids amplified sock drawers more often than not.

However, if you had one channel to amplify 500 Hz and a separate channel to amplify 2,000 Hz, it would give you what you need in each one and sound natural and give you what you need for better understanding and just right volume. That is the beauty of having more channels... it sounds more natural and gives you what you need much better. This way, you actually want to wear them.

Now, all that being said, you have, of course, many more pitches/frequencies in an audiogram involved than just two. There are ten pitches/frequencies that can be tested on an audiogram, so anything up to ten or twelve channels makes sense. I've even seen 16, which is reasonable, if there are harsh drops in hearing at some pitches to make that smoother, but some claim to have 22 or more! Why would you need more channels than you know how to amplify (as in know how much gain to give at each pitch)?? Well, that's a good question, isn't it? It is a selling point. It is to "ooohh" and "aaahhh" you into spending the big bucks or purchase your loyalty with channels. Any more than 12 really, unless you have a steep drop in your hearing, the sound quality does not appear to change or improve in most listeners. Some very discriminatory listeners (my dear engineers or skilled musicians, for instance) will notice a slight difference in sound quality or comfort, but very few.

Now, what I think is more important is how many bands I have control over. A "band", in terms of hearing aids, is a separately adjustable frequency region that I can program however I want (hopefully). In my humble opinion, how many bands I can adjust for people, regardless of how many channels the instrument has, is more important to me. It allows me to make very specific changes when adjusting the aids for the comfort and preference of the individual.

I have seen some hearing aids that claim to have 22 channels and have only 6 bands. This to me is ridiculous, because it bundles the channels for me to program and will sound the same as an aid with 6 channels by the time you're through reprogramming it. So, a more important question is, "How many individual frequencies can you program?"

Ideally, a 12-16 channel hearing aid with 8-10 separate adjustable bands is going to sound wonderful. That being said, if programmed correctly, an 8 channel, 8 band hearing aid sound pretty good too for much less money. I hate to see hearing aids where I can only program the low pitches and high pitches independently in a group. This does not properly take advantage of the technology that is out there, and companies that do that are making a lot of money on their pathetic aids.

There are many other aspects of programming a hearing aid, such as compression ratio, kneepoint, headroom, and so on, that your Audiologist understands and will utilize in programming the aids. I won't get into them here, as it won't interest most of you. You can always call me or do some research on these topics.

Two more things I will mention, however, that will make a considerable difference in which hearing aid you might wish to purchase and good questions to ask before you do. The first is feedback control.

"Feedback" is the unwanted re-amplification of the original amplified sound. I'm sure we've all been attacked at some point in our lives by someone holding a microphone that gets too close to the speaker, creating that ear-piercing squeal that about floors you. Well that is because the amplified sound is feeding back into the speaker and being re-amplified over and over, adding to the sound until it maxes out in the obnoxious and painful sound. The same concept holds true in a microscopic sense with hearing aids. If the amplified sound is re-amplified over and over (in a loop, they call it), the squeal is heard, which is actually feedback.

The old fashioned way to eliminate that was to seal off the vent and make the hearing aid or earmold as tight as humanly possible or just lower the high pitches (which is usually what is necessarily amplified the most). The problem with doing that is that you are taking away valuable hearing where you may need it most and your ear can't breathe and you get a muffled or hollow sound to your own voice.

So, onward comes technology, and our options are better now. The newer digital hearing aids have a filter that detects the feedback before it is detectable via phase cancellation. You can look that one up or call me... most people don't care what exactly that means. However, most people are very happy about what it does. Is it perfect? No, absolutely not. Is it better than it's ever been? Yes, absolutely. Some manufacturers, however, do not have this technology and still turn high pitches down and plug up vents to eliminate/reduce feedback. Please do us all a favor and insist on the manufacturers that have the digital phase cancellation for feedback. You will be happier and the rest of us won't have to listen to you squealing down the street.

The second thing I will discuss with you is also very important. It has to do with most people's biggest complaint or problem with having a hearing loss. What it is, you may be asking? Most of you know... it is noise, of course. And what does "noise" mean and why is reducing it so important? Well, I'm glad you asked. "Noise" is typically thought of as any unwanted sound that interferes with any wanted sound, such as speech. However, I will take it one step further... some "noise" is actually wanted. For example, music can be "noise", even though it is often desirable. If music is playing in a movie, TV show, at a restaurant, or while company is talking: it is noise, but while you are appreciating an amazing symphony: it ceases being "noise" and becomes valued and appreciated.

Why is background noise so bothersome? Well, the first reason is that many hearing losses are sloping from normal or mild or even moderate in the low pitches to higher in the mid or high pitches, meaning the hearing is still better in the lower pitches. Noise is most often centered in the lower pitches, so it masks/blocks those low pitches you are usually better at hearing, making you rely more heavily on the higher pitches, which you are usually worse at hearing, so misunderstandings occur more often.

The second reason is that it is naturally harder to hear a certain person talking in the presence of a lot of noise or other people talking. It is funny to me (funny strange, not funny tee hee, ha ha) that people, after getting hearing aids, have these vast, amazing expectations of hearing perfectly in any circumstance with them, even better than they ever heard with normal hearing! Better than Superman!! Through steel!!!

I have normal hearing right now, thank God and knock on wood, and I have difficulty hearing my husband sometimes when he's sitting across from me in a very crowded and noisy restaurant. I'm having him repeat himself often in there. That's just the way it is. Too much sound is very difficult even with normal hearing because the hearing system is so bombarded with too many sounds that differentiation can only happen with constant focus and use of the eyes (as in lip-reading) to assist me and you. Some places are just not conducive to a good conversation. So, if my husband and I want to talk about deep, intellectual or spiritual matters, we go to a quiet restaurant or more often discuss those things at home, where it is quiet (until my toddler wakes up).

So, noise reduction necessarily occurs in hearing aids now. This noise reduction is the main difference between whether your ride will be bumpy or smooth, your listening experience mediocre or fabulous. Unless finances dictate it, please do yourself a favor and get for yourself a hearing aid with noise reduction. That being said, there are three main levels of noise reduction... the more basic hearing aid has mild noise reduction. The midline hearing aid has up to moderate noise reduction. The top-of-the-line hearing aid had up to strong noise reduction. Does that mean it cancels out every noise on the planet? No, absolutely not. And believe it or not, you wouldn't want it too. However, in general, the more noise reduction you have, the better you are going to hear in more situations and the more natural it will sound when you do.

Speaking of noise reduction, insist on dual microphones (which should come automatically with behind the ear (BTE) hearing aids and cannot come in completely in the canal (CIC) hearing aids). Some manufacturers make hearing aids with three mircrophones, which patients report as very similar or identical to two... just a different way to do the same thing. All hearing aids in my office (except for CIC hearing aids, which can't do it because of space limitations) automatically come with directional/two microphones, and I factor that into my price automatically. Why? Because it is really the main way our signal-to-noise ratio improves.

What on earth is a signal to noise ratio? Well, I'm glad you asked. When someone's speaking, that's the signal. When noise is present, that's the noise. When we are trying to communicate at a party or restaurant or just in the presence of noise, we are trying to hear the signal above the noise, so we want an improved signal to noise ratio. This matters because it is how well we can hear people talking to us (meaningful information) over the noise (non-meaningful information).

So, in summary, how smooth your ride is (how comfortable your hearing is) is determined by the noise reduction and directional microphones, feedback reduction, ability to program the hearing aids to be specific for your hearing loss (number of channels **and** bands), and size. That last one is actually a preference and more comfortable because it is what you want, not because the sound changes much with size (although many of my patients with behind-the-ear [BTE] hearing aids generally say the sound is better than in-the-ear [ITE] hearing aids they've worn). These are the main factors, and everything else is generally of negligible importance, at least with the technology available while I am hitting these keys.

Chapter 8
The Insurance Game

If you are employed full time, at least at the time of writing this book, there is a delightful and amazingly helpful resource worthy of your consideration. The Department of Vocational Rehabilitation (generally listed in the "county" section of the governmental pages of the phone book under the "Department of Education"), assists people by providing or helping pay for hearing aids as needed for your job. They are in the business of keeping people employed and assist employed people with hearing disabilities. This is an amazing help to many working people.

If you are eligible for Veteran's benefits, you can call and ask or set up an appointment to see if they will help or pay for hearing aids for you. Ask what the procedure is. Some VA offices want you to get your hearing tested elsewhere and bring the test results in and some want you to schedule an appointment for testing with their own Audiologist. There is usually a waiting period, as is true for most governmental services, but it is well worth the wait if it saves you from completely paying for your hearing aids (or paying for them at all).

For children in school (under the age of 18 usually), there are services available through the county or state in the school, mostly if you fit a certain economic criteria (parents make under a certain amount). You can speak with the county (usually) Educational Audiologist or consult the school liaison or nurse for options. They are generally required to provide an FM system and additional tutoring or classes and sometimes hearing aids (again hit or miss). They will more so through Medicaid, if you are eligible.

However, there are vast quantities of hard of hearing people who are retired or unemployed or part-timers or ineligible for veteran's benefits or vocational rehabilitation's benefits or whose parents make too much money for various reasons. To these people, insurance coverage is rather hit or miss. Often times, patients are just on their own to purchase hearing aids.

For those on Medicare, at this time, there is coverage for the hearing test but no, I repeat **no coverage** for hearing aids through Medicare alone. Many supplemental plans that simply cover what Medicare doesn't cover also do not cover hearing aids. Now, isn't that terrible?! A very necessary thing like hearing aids and it isn't covered by Medicare! I know... it is very wrong. However, that is the case at this time, so we must forge on. I would encourage those annoyed by this fact to write to your congressman or senator and voice your concerns.

I am asked a lot about hearing aid benefits through AARP. At this time, there are plans for a couple certain states (Florida is one of them) to have a hearing aid discount/partial benefit starting December of 2008. Before that, there was no coverage through them. You can call them and check if your state is one that is covered.

Anyway, for those on Medicaid, hearing aid coverage (for a very basic hearing aid or two aids in some states) varies for each state. Some states only cover the aids for patients under 16 or 18, and some only cover one every three or five years, etc. The best thing to do with this coverage is to call your case worker or look online for the hearing aid benefits for your state.

Now, all that being said, there are some insurance plans (whether the primary plan or supplemental to Medicare) that do cover some or most of the hearing aids' cost, and a very few plans who cover it all! The very best idea is to consult your insurance book or call the customer service number on the back (usually) of your insurance card and as for the hearing aid benefits for your insurance plan. A new trend is for insurance companies to give you a discount program, which means you have to go to certain hearing centers specified on the plan and they in turn give you a "discount", but know this: very often this discounted price has been the exact same price as my normal everyday prices. (I'm really not making any friends now!) Regardless, if you call the phone number on the back of your insurance card, there are certain questions you should ask, that I will address a little later.

So, after you get off your two or three-hour conversation with your insurance company (because you had to get through the automated system and wait on hold about an hour on top of that for a live person), you'll have your answer. Yes, it's just that easy!

However, if you don't feel particularly happy about doing all that yourself or can't hear their questions on the automated system, please feel free to call your local Audiologist and ask them to do it for you. They would be happy to help you! That's what we do. Often, we'll know the coverage for the most common plans already and just have to verify your eligibility- however with all the insurances out there, don't count on it!

For those insurance plans that do cover hearing aids, some of the coverage is a few hundred dollars toward hearing aids, and some pays for one hearing aid, and you would have to pay for the other. Other plans pay for both up to a certain amount. In any of them, if there is a difference between what is owed and what the insurance company pays, you pay the difference. For all of them (unless specified), if you want a higher level of technology than they allow, you pay the difference.

I wish I could give you a fairer world, but that is what we have. Many people pay for hearing aids out of pocket. Most Audiologists these days will have payment plans of some sort or accept credit cards (if perchance you happen to have an offer for low or no interest for so many months), which allows you to make payments. However, do be careful of interest rates if you do not pay the minimum monthly amounts per month when it is due.

One thing about insurance these days is important to know. Insurance companies are in the business of making money. With few exceptions, they put their stockholders' interests above that of the patients whose deductibles is funding those interests. In times past, it was not that way, or at least was to a lesser degree. Now, it's a totally different ballgame. There are higher deductibles and copays and patient's responsibility. They often tell you where to go for healthcare, whether you like them or not.

In some states (like mine, for instance) another factor in all this is monopoly insurance middle-men, who people have to be a provider for to bill certain insurance companies. However, if you are within 30 miles of that middle-man's own company, you have to go to their company only. These middle-men end up sharing the insurance payment in exchange for doing some of the middle-men stuff. The person who benefits is the middle-man and the insurance company. If people have transportation issues and cannot drive the 30 miles to the nearest middle-man company, they don't have to provide the hearing aid benefit. If they do find the transportation, the middle-man gets the benefit. Outside of the 30-mile limit, they still get a cut of the action, taking a portion of the insurance payment away from the Audiologist. So, who loses? Of course, the professional and unfortunately the patient.

Another factor is that if one insurance company promises a benefit of, say $500 per hearing aid, often the provider actually only receives $250 and has to "discount" the rest of that. But I can imagine that I am probably the only one who has ever enlightened you about that. Most people don't know the inner workings of the insurance companies. Also, they often take, with few exceptions, 30 **business** days up to 6 months to actually pay the provider. In addition, some insurance companies (in my county, Humana is a big culprit in this) say they cover so much when you call them and then tell you a month after you submit the claim that it is not a covered benefit. Other insurance companies also regularly deny claims the first time for no very good reason at all and make you resubmit them. Then, they can hold onto "their" money longer to get the interest. Enormous insurance and healthcare reforms are necessary, as you probably already know, but that is how it is for now as I write this. So, many Audiologists, to survive, have stopped accepting certain insurance companies or make the patient pay up front and the patient be reimbursed by the insurance company. Now you know why.

Also, when you first get into the Audiologist's office or beforehand, we call to determine your hearing aid benefits. Most people do not know what their hearing aid benefit is, if there is any. It helps if people look it up or over before coming in for the visit, so they know what they're looking at. The phone number is in your provider book or on the back (generally) of your insurance card (or call your case worker, if applicable). The long-awaited intelligent questions to ask are:

1. What is my effective date?
2. Do I have a hearing aid benefit?
3. If yes, is it for one or both ears?
4. Also if yes, what is the maximum allowable per aid?
5. How often am I eligible for this benefit?
6. Do I need a medical clearance for hearing aids?
7. Do I need a physician referral?
8. Is there a copay involved?
9. Is there a separate deductible **or** what is my remaining deductible before hearing aid coverage?
10. Does the Audiologist have to be in network or can I go to anyone?
11. If they have to be in network, what Audiologists can I go to?

That pretty much takes care of the intelligent insurance questions. Now, be sure to write down the answers... don't rely on your memory because that is a lot of numbers and things to remember, and it's best not to put yourself through all that. Not all questions are needed, but sometimes they are. When in doubt, ask anyway... it certainly won't hurt anything.

Let me be so bold as to say that if you ask these questions and bring in the answers to your Audiologist for your appointment, you will be so much appreciated that you won't even know what to do with the warmth generated by the staff! I say this because a lot of time is taken up by us asking these questions, because many, if not most, patients have no idea what their hearing aid benefits are.

That being said, if you can not or do not know how to make that call or it is too difficult for you for any reason, please don't feel you must. We can... it just takes a little time. It takes time whether you do it yourself or we do it for you. It is a royal pain to get through the automated systems of these insurance companies, and hearing aid benefits to this day have never been addressed in the automated system... you have to muddle through it to get to a live person. And that is indeed a daunting task and not for the timid of heart. I think they do that on purpose to discourage you from checking. Of course, that last sentence is just my own biased opinion.

One insurance company is certain. At the time of writing this book, Medicare does **not** cover hearing aids. Let me repeat that, Medicare does **not** cover hearing aids. They cover hearing tests but not a penny toward hearing aids. So don't bother calling them... I don't see that changing, although Audiologists have been fighting for it for years.

All other insurance companies' plans are often different on a state by state basis. For instance, as of this writing, Blue Cross Blue Shield of Florida does not cover hearing aids, but Blue Cross Blue Shield of Michigan sometimes does, depending on the plan. Right now, there is a bill on the floor to give a $500 per ear tax credit for hearing aid purchases, but I'm not sure how that will turn out, so call an accountant or look online to find out before you hold me to that.

To save time, you can ask your Audiologist if he/she knows through experience if certain insurance companies cover hearing aids or not. If they don't know, then you or they can call and find out. Don't take them not knowing as a sign that they are inexperienced or unknowledgeable, though, because there are hundreds of insurance companies and even more variations of each plan. Each plan is often different and each state is different. And some states are very different, if you know what I mean! Yeah, I'm just kidding there.

Chapter 9
Do These Aids Make Me Look Old?

So, here is an interesting and loaded question... "Do these aids make me look old?" Well, let's explore that a little. First of all, if you have been paying attention to what you've been reading up to now, let me just remind you that even babies and children sometimes need to wear hearing aids. If you have **not** been paying attention... why not? Hmmmm?

Well, other than that point, let me give you a scenario. You walk into a small dinner party at a friend's house. There are two particular people before you that you've met before. One gentleman, say mid-sixties, has salt and pepper hair, is clean cut, and is actively involved in a normal conversation with the host. Upon further examination, because you naturally have a great attention to details, you realize that that gentleman is wearing hearing aids. At least you think that's what they are. It's hard to tell for sure, though, because they're so small... just a tiny piece behind his ears the same color as his hair and a small clear tube going into his ears.

Another gentleman, say also mid-sixties, has brown hair (because he dies it), is also clean cut, and is also actively involved in a conversation with the host's wife. What is different about his conversation is that he is speaking very loudly. Not only that, but he is laughing at inappropriate times and brushes it off with a little additional laugh when he realizes it. Also, he seems to be asking her to repeat herself quite often and is misunderstanding her answers. She is trying to be patient, but her body language says that she is uncomfortable.

Now, in that scenario, which of these gentlemen look older? More importantly, which of them look more intelligent? Now, if I were the person walking in, I would certainly have observed that the first gentleman, who actually was wearing hearing aids, was certainly taking a proactive, intelligent action towards being a generous conversationalist and partaker of the conversation. I say generous because in giving himself better hearing, he also was giving his listener the opportunity to communicate with him. And after all, we are all created to socialize. How much happier would his wife be at home also, how less stressful her conversations with her husband, how much he must love her to wear the hearing aids for them both!

The second gentleman, on the other hand, would appear to be either in denial of a hearing loss so evident to everyone around him, which makes him look unintelligent, or too vain to wear them, thinking wearing them would make him look old or hard of hearing. Now, does he not look selfish also? I bet his wife, who looks fatigued, is happy to finally be out talking to other people she **can** associate with without getting a stress headache or feeling unable to easily communicate with her own beloved (and less beloved by the day) husband.

Now, please understand that this scenario was not intended to make anyone feel guilty, but to explore this faulty idea of hearing aids making anyone look old. I believe, and believed long before I went into the profession of Audiology, that people who wear hearing aids are intelligent and high tech and lovers of life and socialization. I think most people believe that. I think the bigger problem, truth be told, is that in order to partake in a solution, you have to first admit that there is a problem that requires one. That, I believe, is a huge leap and the heart of the matter.

The second aspect of the looks of these hearing aids is that these days they are so cosmetically appealing, that vanity is almost a non-issue these days. The tiny little behind the ear hearing aids (like Resound's

Dot or Be series or Widex's Passion series, and the list goes on and on), are so small that most people don't even see them at all. If people can hardly see them and they don't jump out at you, what does it matter to even the vainest of people whether you wear them or not?

I think that it goes back to the statement that it is more often the wearer alone that holds the unfair stereotype that wearing hearing aids means you're old. Get rid of that. It is untrue and extremely unfair. People don't really care that anyone's wearing hearing aids- half the time they don't know they're even being worn-, but they **do** care when they aren't being able to communicate properly with the hard of hearing patient who consistently misunderstands but won't do anything about it.

Ya know what I've always found funny? Well, I'm glad you asked. Some patients are eager, no excited about telling me and everyone they meet that they just had a colonoscopy or urologist appointment or "fascinating" weird cyst growth or "interesting" fungal infection in their toenails and all the exciting details of those physician visits/procedures. And yet, they are horrified when they are told that their hearing has worsened to the point that hearing aids are recommended. Wait a minute! You didn't have a problem with all those other disgusting things to be voiced to the world at large, but you are horrified to wear very clean, intelligent hearing aids??? You thought it was funny too, didn't you? Come on, admit it. I heard you. Ha!

So, to answer the question if the hearing aids make you look old... the resounding answer is **NO!!!** (Which, by the way, is the exact same answer to the similar question, "Does this dress make me look fat?", regardless of what you want to answer.) In fact, wearing them makes you look good in many ways. You look smart, sociable, generous, loving, kind, pleasant to converse with, extravagant in some instances, and relatable. No, not more handsome, but not less handsome either. For heaven's sake, look at all the wackos- no offense, wackos- running around with humungous blue tooth ear things hanging on their ears!! They think they look cool and high tech!! Tee-hee! They paid sometimes a fortune for those things and are going to sport them, by golly!

Chapter 10
The Light at the End of the Tunnel

So, I hope you have learned everything you need to know to make an informed decision to be tested by an Audiologist, understand the test results, know something about insurance that might help, understand about hearing aids and differences in hearing aid technologies, understand the value of the hearing aids and reasonable price expectations, and know that it is not going to make you look old or dorky or senile, etc. to wear them. That was my goal.

There are millions of people in this world that have hearing loss great enough to warrant hearing aid use. You are not alone, if you fit into that category. You also have better technology in the hearing aids available to you than anyone has that gone before you! That's huge!

There are great people who wear hearing aids. There are beautiful people who wear hearing aids. There are butt ugly people who wear hearing aids. There are babies who wear hearing aids. There are dogs who wear hearing aids (I wouldn't doubt it).

I want you to know that there is hope for those who are hard of hearing. It is not a sin, a curse, a lost cause, a reason for depression, etc. to have a hearing loss anymore. It is a fact of life. It is treatable. Hearing aids are a viable, albeit expensive, treatment. They can change your life.

They all come (state-mandated) with a 30-day trial period, so you can always return them within the 30 days with only a $150 for one or $200 for two penalty if you do return them. So, the worst that can happen is that you're out $200 max, but trying can change your life.

If you have any further questions, please feel free to email me or check out my website for further clarification or any of the many resources listed below (websites and books). Please don't believe everything you hear, but do believe me. I have nothing to profit from lying to you.

A hearing loss is not the end of the world, but in our hearing world, it is difficult to participate in all it has to offer without correcting that hearing loss. So, please enjoy the experience of wearing properly fitted hearing aids.

And by all means, during the trial period, if you are not happy with the hearing aids or person who fitted you, **GIVE THEM BACK** and find someone else who is more competent. It is your right and responsibility to do so. And even more importantly, if you find someone who is unethical in their practices or attempts to stall you into keeping them past the 30-day trial, not only leave immediately, but also do someone else a favor and report them to the Better Business Bureau (which is also a good place to check before going to anyone to begin with). Most people remain silent and just chalk it up as a loss, but these people will remain out there to do it again to someone else unless held responsible for their actions.

If you do meet a bad apple or got taken in by a dishonest hearing aid specialist, please don't beat yourself up about it or be frustrated. These people are very convincing and well-versed in what they do. And some hearing aid specialists are great... I would just **prefer** or recommend you go to an Audiologist.

The thing is, as you know, there are good and bad in every profession. There are good and bad physicians, good and bad hair stylists (yes, I've been victimized before by one!), good and bad mechanics, good and bad surgeons (unfortunately), and you never know which they are until they do something that lets you know. The same is true of Audiologists. If you are unhappy with your aids, go back and let them know. Give them a chance or two to fix it (most digital fittings take 2-3 visits before the sound is perfect). If they don't, return it and go somewhere else.

The key is to not give up. Don't give up on hearing aids. Don't give up on participating in the conversation. Don't give up on going out or attending parties, weddings, church, receptions, or funerals. Don't give up on your family or friends that love you and want to talk to you. Most people with untreated hearing loss will start to withdraw and hibernate to some extent, which increases depression, loneliness, and isolation.

You can again participate in life. Hearing aids may be the answer to get you in the social aspects of life again. A hearing loss is treatable! That is my answer. That is our hope! Don't give up... just get hearing! Happy listening!!!!

Resources
Riding This Horse to Death

1. www.audiologyonline.org
2. www.lakelandhearing.com
3. www.asha.org
4. www.trydotbyresound.com
5. www.mygnresound.com
6. www.widex.com
7. www.phonak.com
8. www.siemens.com
9. www.starkey.com
10. www.rexton.com
11. www.betterhearing.com
12. www.betterbusinessbureau.com
13. Hearing Loss & Hearing Aids.

www.ingramcontent.com/pod-product-compliance
Lightning Source LLC
Chambersburg PA
CBHW061803280526
45787CB00003BA/1462